Homoeopathic Remedies for Children

PHYLLIS SPEIGHT

Homoeopathic Remedies for Children

Health Science Press
The C. W. Daniel Company Ltd
1 Church Path, Saffron Walden, Essex, England

First published in Great Britain by
The C. W. Daniel Company Limited
1 Church Path, Saffron Walden
Essex, England

Reprinted 1986, 1989 (twice)

ISBN 0 85207 158 2

Set in 10pt Melior 2pt leaded by MFK Typesetting Ltd, Saffron Walden
and printed by Hillman Printers (Frome) Ltd,
Frome, Somerset

CONTENTS

PREFACE

No mother likes to see her child unwell or suffering. Children can change from being well and rushing around one minute to being off-colour and exhibiting symptoms the next; and then medicines like aspirin or antibiotics are frequently administered to give relief.

More and more people are becoming concerned about the effects of drugs, particularly in relation to children. Many mothers telephone me to ask for help and advice because they do not wish to give their children drugs which have been prescribed.

There is an alternative in homoeopathy. Our medicines are safe and never, ever cause side-effects. When the correct remedy is chosen spectacular things happen in many cases of acute diseases and there is no reason why parents cannot use homoeopathic remedies effectively if they will give a little time to understand and study the following pages.

I hope this book will bring many people to homoeopathic prescribing for the simple, every-day, acute troubles from which many children suffer.

Phyllis Speight
Devon, 1983

TO PARENTS

Please Study This – It is Important

Homoeopathy is a complete system of medicine which has been in use for over 200 years. It is safe, cannot cause any side effects and is curative – in other words it does not suppress symptoms.

But homoeopathic remedies must be matched to the symptoms of the child. There are no specifics in Homoeopathy.

Let me give you an instance of what I mean. If your child swallows some berries of Deadly Nightshade (Belladonna) he would develop a temperature, a very hot, red face, dilated pupils and probably a very sore throat. If the child suddenly develops what we might call a fever with these similar symptoms, then Belladonna in homoeopathic form would cure him quickly because 'Like cures like'.

Obviously many remedies have common symptoms like sneezing, vomiting, shivering etc., but each remedy has a set of what we call 'characteristic' symptoms which are not in others and so differentiate one remedy from another. One of the characteristic symptoms of Belladonna is 'very red, hot face – the heat can be felt before the hand touches the skin'.

Although we have over 2000 remedies in our materia medicas I have chosen just twenty-five in order not to muddle you too much at the beginning and these are medicines which we use over and over again for children.

I have set these out in an order which I feel will be more simple for you to understand than the schema in our materia medicas.

At the beginning I have given the 'Characteristic symptoms' followed by any outstanding symptoms found in children.

It will help tremendously if you study these symptoms and memorize some of them because then you will recognise them in your children when they are sick.

Following the Characteristics I have given a list of acute conditions that the remedy has cured – for instance under Aconite (which is one of the first remedies that comes to mind when any child is ill because one of it's Characteristics is 'sudden beginning of illness with fever and anxiousness' which is so common) I have listed Chicken-pox, Colds, Cough, Croup, Diarrhoea, Ear-troubles, Excitement effects of, Fever, Headache, Influenza, Insomnia, Measles, Mumps, Nervous troubles, Stomach troubles, Toothache, and Throat troubles. If the little patient is exhibiting the symptoms given under any of these headings, then Aconite will help.

It does not matter what we call a disease – if the symptoms of Aconite correspond to the symptoms of the child he will be cured and the interesting thing is we do not know what has been aborted because a sudden rise in temperature with fever can advance to bronchitis, pneumonia, influenza and many other troubles; this is what is so satisfying about Homoeopathy, we know that the correct remedy will cure the patient with no suppression of any kind.

I must stress, however, that Aconite and the other twenty-four remedies, cover a much wider field and symptoms of Aconite, for instance, fill ten pages in Hering's Condensed Materia Medica which is not, by any means, a full one.

Following the twenty-five remedies you will find a Repertory of Characteristic Mind Symptoms. This comprises the mind symptoms from all the remedies in alphabetical order.

Then follows a list of General Characteristics compiled in the same way and then two lists of Modalities that make the condition better or worse. A general Repertory follows for each trouble, again in alphabetical order.

I have tried to keep this as simple as possible. There are many books on Homoeopathy which you can obtain to gain more knowledge as time goes on.

Obviously in the scope of this small book the number of remedies is limited for every complaint and this applies especially to the infectious diseases. I have included a list of books for further reading and study at the end which will help to solve some of these problems.

Once you have got the basic idea that you prescribe the remedy to match the symptoms of your child you can add to your knowledge by studying more medicines.

HOW TO FIND THE CORRECT REMEDY

When seeking the remedy for the sick child it is necessary to write down the symptoms. He may be able to answer questions as to how he feels, where the pain is, what the pain is like and what makes it better, or worse.

But you must learn to be very observant. Is the child lethargic or restless; is he sweating, if so where particularly; does he want to be nursed; is he frightened or anxious and so on.

In addition the modalities are most important and so also is the cause, if known.

The more you study the twenty-five remedies and the Repertory of symptoms the more familiar you will become with what Homoeopathy is all about.

With the list of symptoms you may be able to spot the remedy quickly. If not you should consult the Repertory under the heading of the particular trouble and then the list of modalities. You should then consider one or two remedies and study them with the aid of the Materia Medica. The most appropriate one should be administered.

Always remember that the most important symptoms appear under 'Characteristics' and if you can find three of these you can prescribe with confidence, providing they are marked in the child. You can sit safely on a three legged stool but you will fall over on two legs!

The more you study the twenty-five remedies and the Repertory of symptoms the more familiar you will become with what Homoeopathy is all about.

THE 25 REMEDIES AND ABBREVIATIONS

Aconitum Napellus	Acon.
Antimonium Crudum	Ant. c.
Antimonium Tartaricum	Ant. t.
Argentum Nitricum	Arg. n.
Arsenicum Album	Ars. alb.
Baryta Carb	Bar. c.
Belladonna	Bell.
Bryonia	Bry.
Calcarea Carbonica	Calc. c.
Calcarea Phosphorica	Calc. p.
Capsicum	Caps.
Causticum	Caust.
Chamomilla	Cham.
Cinchona Officinalis	China.
Gelsemium	Gels.
Hepar Sulphuris	Hep. s.
Ignatia	Ign.
Lycopodium	Lyc.
Mercurius	Merc.
Natrum Muriaticum	Nat.m.
Nux Vomica	Nux. v.
Phosphorus	Phos.
Pulsatilla	Puls.
Silicea	Sil.
Sulphur	Sulph.

HOMOEOPATHIC REMEDIES

Homoeopathic remedies are prepared in a special way by Homoeopathic Chemists and should always be purchased from a reputable firm.

They are sensitive and should be kept in a drawer or cupboard away from sunlight and strong smelling perfumes or soaps etc., and they should not be taken directly after cleaning the teeth with a flavoured toothpaste.

Pills or tablets should be handled as little as possible – usually they can be shaken into the cap of the bottle or box and popped into the mouth.

One pill or tablet is sufficient for one dose. Put one or the other under the tongue where it will dissolve – do NOT wash it down with water. If the child is too young to cope with pills or tablets then put two or three of either in a quarter of a tumblerful of water, stir well and give one teaspoonful as a dose.

In acute troubles remedies may be given frequently in the 6th or 12th potencies – half-hourly if necessary but usually one or two hourly is adequate – this depends entirely how severe the condition is. The golden rule is that as improvement develops the time between doses must be widened and the medicine stopped as soon as the patient is much better – remedies continue to work in the system for some time after the last dose has been taken.

If similar symptoms return then the remedy may be repeated but if new symptoms appear then a different remedy must be found to match them.

If after a day the patient is not improving another must be found to match the symptoms more accurately. Do NOT change the remedy too quickly. This emphasizes the importance of finding the correct remedy.

If there is no sign of improvement or the child gets worse then a doctor must be consulted at once.

ACONITUM NAPELLUS

Characteristics:

Acute, sudden and violent invasion with fever.
Sudden beginning of illness where there is fever with intense anxiety and restlessness and fear. Can vomit with fear.
Symptoms appear after exposure to dry cold winds.
There is much tension, *Aconite* has a calming effect.
Skin hot and dry.
Thirst with fever.
Better open air.
Worse warm room; night, around midnight.

The following characteristics are often found in children who need this remedy:
Always restless, anxious and frightened.

Aconite can be used in the following complaints providing the symptoms agree:

Chicken Pox: First stage of initial fever with anxiety and restlessness.

Colds: First sneeze or shiver especially after exposure to dry cold. Frequent sneezing with dropping of clear hot water from nostrils. Worse in stuffy atmosphere.

Cough: After exposure to dry, cold wind. Short, dry cough, wakens child from sleep, also when entering a warm room.

Croup: Aconite, Hepar sulph, Spongia, Hepar sulph, Spongia at 2–4 hourly intervals in that order.

Diarrhoea: Watery stools brought on by dry, cold wind or fright.

Ear Troubles: Sudden, after chills or exposure to cold. Ear red, hot and painful. Better warm applications.

Excitement; Effects of: Brought about by fear and restlessness.

Fever: Dry, burning skin. Face red but pale on sitting up. Great thirst, restlessness, agitation. Worse in evening and around midnight.

Headache: Sudden and violent. As if tight band were around head. Throbbing in temples moving from one side to the other. Restlessness, anxiety, thirsty.

Influenza: Sudden onset of fever with chilliness, great restlessness and anxiety.

Insomnia: Kept awake by fear or panic. Sleeplessness from shock or fright. Restless tossing.

Measles: Fever, catarrh before rash appears, eyes red, barking cough, itching burning skin. Restless, anxious, frightened.

Mumps: Fever, anxiety, restlessness.

Nervous Troubles: Extreme anxiety, impatience, fears. Cannot stand pain, noise, music. Confused thoughts and ideas.

Stomach Troubles: Vomiting from fright.

Toothache: Pain after filling.

Throat Troubles: Very dry with burning and tingling. Swallowing causes pain. Desires cold water. From exposure to dry, cold wind.

ANTIMONIUM CRUDUM

Characteristics:

Thickly coated white, very white tongue.
Derangements from overloading the stomach, especially with fat foods, nausea.
Finger nails grow in splits with horny spots.
Corns and callosities on soles of feet.
Child cannot bear to be looked at.
Fitful, cross.
Feverish conditions at night.
Cannot bear heat of sun.
Exhausted in warm weather.
Worse heat and heat of sun and radiated heat.
Worse cold bathing.

The following characteristics are often found in children who need this remedy:

Fat, irritable, sulky and peevish; the more attention they get the more peevish they become.

They will cry if anyone looks at them and are worse if soothed.

They sometimes suffer from night terrors.

They are impressionable and sensitive and easily upset emotionally, when they will burst into tears.

Any stress or strain makes them very pale and they are liable to faint.

They are clumsy children with jerky movements.

Antimonium crudum can be used in the following complaints providing the symptoms agree:

Extremities: Aches and pains from taking a cold bath or getting wet in the rain.

Cough: Worse coming into a warm room from the cold with burning sensation in chest.

Diarrhoea: Often follows upset stomach, worse in summer heat, when stools are often partly solid and partly liquid. Nausea, vomiting, diarrhoea worse heat of sun.

Ear Troubles: Moist eruption behind ears.

Extremities: Aches and pains from taking a cold bath or getting wet in the rain.

Eye Troubles: Redness round the eyes.

Stomach Troubles: Worse overeating, especially fats, with nausea, feels he will not be better until he has vomited. If accompanied by *very* white tongue this is the first remedy to think of. Acid foods upset. Constant belching.

ANTIMONIUM TARTARICUM

Characteristics:

Great weakness, lassitude.
Drowsiness, debility and sweat.
Sleepiness or sleeplessness.
Great accumulation of mucus in air passages with much rattling and inability to raise it.
Nausea, vomiting, with loss of appetite.
Pallor. Pale sunken face.
Lack of thirst.
Irritability.
Worse evening; from lying down at night; from warmth; in damp, cold weather.
Better sitting erect; from bringing up wind and expectoration.

The following characteristics are often found in children:
Child wants to be carried yet cries if touched.
Will not let you feel their pulse.
They are apprehensive, frightened and restless.

Antimonium Tartaricum can be used in the following complaints providing symptoms agree:

Asthma. Difficulty in breathing, shortness of breath, desires to sit upright. Bronchial tubes seem full of mucus but none comes up.

Chicken Pox: In early stages. Eruption slow in coming out. Often with bronchitis. Patient drowsy, perspires freely. Nausea. Child peevish but likes company.

Cough: Loose cough without expectoration, compels patient to sit up. Much rattling mucus very difficult to get up. Mucus sticky, white, thick. Coughing and gaping consecutively especially in children with crying and dozing, twitching of face. Pain in chest or larynx. Breathing difficult. Nausea and vomiting with cough.

Croup: Advanced stages. Face cold, bluish with cold perspiration. Unable to dislodge mucus. Respiration very difficult, shrill or whistling. Difficult to expand chest.

Stomach Troubles: Vomiting with violent straining and sweat on forehead. Continuous nausea, vomiting and diarrhoea. Green, tough, watery mucus followed by great drowsiness and prostration, coldness and cold sweat.

Whooping cough: Cough preceded by crying or after eating or drinking or when getting warm in bed. Rattling cough, bronchial tubes seem full of mucus but none is expectorated. Nausea and vomiting of large amounts of mucus with cold sweat on forehead.

ARGENTUM NITRICUM

Characteristics:

Fear, anxiety, apprehension regarding future events.
Funks examinations.
Fears failure. Tummy turns over.
Irrational thoughts and imaginations.
Impulsive, does things in a hurry, walks fast.
Claustrophobia.
Looking from heights causes giddiness, looking up at high buildings also causes trouble. When in a threatre or other gathering seeks a seat which will enable him to make a quick exit or escape.
Dreads crowds.
Irresistible desire for sugar and sweet things which aggravate and cause diarrhoea.
Worse heat, feeling of suffocation in a warm room, wants cold air.

The following characteristics are often found in children:
Child can be emaciated, looking old and wrinkled.
Can get very worked up before doing anything new, going to school for the first time etc.

Argentum Nitricum can be used in the following complaints providing symptoms agree:

Colds: Itching of nose. Whitish pus with clots of blood. Thick tenacious mucus causes hawking.

Diarrhoea: Stool green, often like chopped spinach; expelled with spluttering. Much flatus. Worse night, after midnight, sweet things.

Headache: Better by binding something tightly around head. Head feels enlarged. One sided pressure pain. Worse mental effort, violent movement.

Nervous Troubles: Fear of heights, crowds, water. Claustrophobia. Apprehension before an examination, speech, driving test, etc.

Stomach Troubles: Craving for sweets and sugar which worsen the condition. Belching after every meal, which does not relieve. Stomach feels as if wind would cause it to burst.

Throat Troubles: Uvula dark red. Thick, tenacious mucus causes much hawking. Sensation of splinter in throat when swallowing. Rawness, soreness, scraping in throat causing hawking and coughing. Voice rough from using it too much.

ARSENICUM ALBUM

Characteristics:

Great prostration yet marked restlessness from anxiety and fear.

Moves from one bed to another or moves around the bed.

Fear – fright – worry.

Burning pains better by heat but patient always wants the head kept cool.

Discharges burn.

Great thirst for small quantities at frequent intervals.

Fastidious, hates disorder.

Better warmth, except head, loves and craves heat.

Worse at night, after midnight, 1 to 3 a.m., cold air, wet weather, cold drinks, cold applications.

The following characteristics are often found in children who need this remedy:

Very easily frightened, nervy and highly strung; afraid of being alone, going out alone, of the dark.

They will cling to mother from fear rather than from affection.

They suffer from night terrors, are very restless in bed or they will go into mother's bed.

They are very tidy children and will put their toys away when they have finished playing with them, they are unhappy in disorder.

At meal times they do not like sticky hands and if they spill anything they are most upset because they cannot bear any mess.

Arsenicum album can be used in the following complaints providing the symptoms agree:

21

Abscess: Burning and stabbing pains better by heat. Restlessness. Worse after midnight.

Asthma: Breathing worse from 1 to 2 a.m. with great debility and burning in chest, unable to lie down. Worse cold air, motion. Better bending forward, applied heat and hot drinks.

Colds: With thin watery, excoriating discharge. Nose feels stopped up, much sneezing without relief. Throat burning.

Cough: Wheezing respiration; frothy mucus, difficulty in breathing. Worse from midnight to 2 a.m. Restlessness and anxiety.

Dandruff: Dry scurf.

Fever: Fearful and restless. Burning pains better from warmth. Thirsty for frequent sips of water. Worse after midnight. Feels hot and cold alternately.

Hay Fever: Violent sneezing. Tickle inside nose not relieved by sneezing. Profuse watery discharge burns lip. Burning in eyes. Worse change in weather. Restlessness.

Headache: Better by cold air and cold applications. Periodical burning pains with restlessness.

Influenza: Streaming eyes and nose, chilliness and great prostration. Extreme mental restlessness and distress.

Insomnia: Sleepless after midnight. Very restless cannot keep still in bed, often gets out of bed. Is usually anxious.

Ptomaine Poisoning: Vomits and stool are simultaneous.

Stomach Upsets: Cannot bear the sight or smell of food. Great thirst, drinks much but little at a time. Burning pains soon after food. Feeling of weight in stomach. Retching with vomiting causing exhaustion with coldness. Better warm drinks after vomiting.

BARYTA CARB.

Characteristics:

Memory deficient; forgets in the middle of a speech.
Great mental and bodily weakness.
Childishness in old people.
Sadness – dejection of spirits.
Timid, bashful, cowardly.
Dread of strangers.
Irresolute – constantly changing his mind.
Chilly people, need much clothing.
All symptoms are worse after eating.

The following characteristics are often found in children who need this remedy:
Backward, retarded children, both physically and mentally.
Slow to talk and walk.
Child cannot be taught, he cannot remember, is inattentive.
Often physically undersized. Emaciated but has large abdomen.
Very timid and shy.
Does not want to play with other children and is happier in familiar surroundings.

Baryta Carb. can be used in the following complaints providing symptoms agree:

Colds: Develop after becoming chilled or from cold air. Nose runs and upper lip becomes swollen. Scurf under nose. Takes cold very easily.

Coughs: Chronic with swollen glands and enlarged tonsils; worse after slightest cold. Nightly cough, chest full of mucus. Spasmodic cough excited by tickling and toughness in throat, worse evening until midnight, cold air.

Ear Troubles: Thick crust on and behind ears. Itching in ears.

Eye Troubles: Inflamed.

Extremities: Feel cold and clammy with offensive sweat.

Fever: Chill and chilliness better external warmth. Chill alternating with heat evening and night. Thirsty. Debilitating night sweats.

Headache: Dry scurf or moist crusts, itchy and burning. Sensitive to cold.

Throat Troubles: Tonsils inflame, swell and suppurate on every exposure to cold. Smarting in throat when swallowing, worse from empty swallowing; throat sore to touch. Sensation as of a plug in the throat. Worse swallowing solids. Catarrh runs down the back of throat. Throat affections after checked foot-sweat. Liable to tonsillitis after every slight cold or suppressed foot-sweat. The range of this remedy is not wide but indications are very definite.

BELLADONNA

Characteristics:

Heat, redness, throbbing, burning violent.
Acute local inflammations with sudden onset.
Fevers with dry, hot, burning skin, heat can be felt before hand touches it.
Very red flushed face.
Pupils dilated.
Sudden rise in temperature.
Restlessness from excitement.
Mental states which can go on to delirium.
Throbbing in head.

The following characteristics are often found in children:
Often have light hair and fine complexions.
Young full-blooded people with fevers.
Child gets into very excitable moods and is easily brought to tears.

Belladonna can be used in the following complaints providing symptoms agree:

Abscess: Swelling bright red, burning and throbbing, tender. Worse cold air or draught.

Chicken Pox: Headache severe, flushed face, hot skin, drowsiness, inability to sleep.

Colds: Violent onset, not much discharge; nose swollen, sore, red, hot. Throat sore; hoarse with painful dryness of larynx. Face hot, flushed, burning with violent headache. Very thirsty.

25

Cough: Tickling, dry cough, worse at night; in violent paroxysms; great dryness of larynx. Head feels as if it is bursting.

Ear Troubles: Sudden digging, throbbing pain often in right ear. Dry, flushed face. Burning skin. Restlessness. Worse least jar. Better heat.

Excitement, Effect of: Headache.

Fever: Sudden onset. Face very red, high temperature, strong and rapid pulse. Skin burning hot. General sweating. Little or no thirst.

Headache: Bursting, throbbing, head hot. Pain especially forehead, worse least jar, lying down, stooping. Better pressure; sitting up; bending head back; keeping head warm after having hair under dryer and going out in cold. Pain comes on and ceases abruptly.

Mumps: Inflammation of right parotid gland with bright redness; glowing red face, violent shooting pains.

Stomach Troubles: Colic. Better bending forward.

Sunstroke: Burning, dry hot skin. Dilated pupils. Strong pulse.

Throat: Tonsils inflamed, bright red. Throat dry with great burning. Raw and sore looks very raw and shining. Constant urging to swallow, feels as if he would choke if he did not swallow. Feels constricted; congested, angry looking. Worse at night.

Toothache: Throbbing with dry mouth. Gumboil.

Whooping Cough: Child often starts to cry before coughing comes on, sometimes with stomach pains. Spasms of coughing until a little mucus is raised then throat gets dryer and dryer and coughing starts all over again, spasm often ends with whooping.

Worms: is a remedy to be thought of.

BRYONIA

Characteristics:

Complaints develop slowly.
Patient very irritable, do not cross a Bryonia patient, it makes him worse.
Pains are stabbing, stitching, worse for motion.
Great thirst for copious draughts at long intervals.
Dryness of mucous membranes from lips to rectum.
Faintness when sitting up in bed.
Better lying on painful side, pressure, rest, cold things.
Worse slightest motion of any kind. In a damp climate Bryonia is one of the most frequently used remedies.

The following characteristics are often found in children:

They dislike to be carried or raised up.

Bryonia can be used in the following complaints providing symptoms agree:

Colds: Travel down to chest. Symptoms slow to develop, much sneezing, eyes red and water, nasal discharge watery. Lips cracked, lips, mouth and throat dry.

Constipation: Stools hard and dry as if burnt. Much thirst, mouth, lips and tongue very dry.

Cough: Dry and hard with stitches in chest, makes child sit up in bed. Worse going into warm room; worse movement.

Diarrhoea: Much purging early morning, from sour fruit or drinking cold water when overheated.

Headache: Pain bursting, splitting, worse motion, even moving the eyes. Frontal headache. Frontal sinuses may be involved.

Influenza: Painful cough, pain in throat and chest. Thirst with dry mouth and lips. Wants to lie quite still. Aches all over. Headache.

Insomnia: Wakes screaming from anxious dreams.

Measles: High temperature. Dull look with swollen face. Headache. Mouth dry with thirst for cold water. Feels cold but wants air. Cough caused by chest involvement.

Stomach Upsets: Distress in pit of stomach soon after food; nausea and faintness on attempting to sit up. Waterbrash, biliousness, heartburn. Thirst for large quantities but warm drinks are vomited. Colic worse movement, touch or pressure, heat. Child may be motionless on back with knees drawn up.

Whooping Cough: Child coughs immediately after eating and drinking, vomits and then returns to the table to continue the meal. Dry, spasmodic cough shaking the whole body, makes child spring out of bed.

CALCAREA CARBONICA

Characteristics:

Fat, flabby, fair, faint, fearful.
There are so many fears for the future, misfortune, health etc.
Hand is soft, cool and boneless, gives you the shivers to shake hands with Calcaria.
Everything smells sour – stool, sweat, urine. Taste is sour.
Glands are often enlarged.
Slow in movement.
Craves eggs and indigestible things like chalk, earth, raw potatoes.
Feels better when constipated.
Profuse cold, sour sweat about head.
Sweats even in a cold room.
Feet feel as if wearing cold, damp stockings.
Great sensitivity to cold and cold damp weather; dreads open air, at the same time cannot bear the sun.
Breathless – walking slowly up a slight hill can bring on sweating and breathlessness.
Better after breakfast. Drawing up limbs. Loosening garments. In the dark. Lying on back. From rubbing. Dry, warm weather. Worse on waking. Morning. After midnight. Bathing. Working in water. Full moon. New Moon. Mental and physical exertion. Stooping. Pressure of clothes. Open air. Cold air. *Cold, wet weather.* Letting limbs hang down.

The following characteristics are often found in children:
They are fair, fat, chilly, lethargic and sweaty; late in walking.
There is fatness without fitness; quantity but not quality.
The baby is fat, podgy, smiling sweetly but does not make any attempt to move.

Stamina is low so they cannot keep up anything for very long, either physically or mentally. Sluggish physically and mentally. They are quite happy to sit and do nothing or very little. They are bad at games.
Slow in walking and cutting teeth.
Typical rickets children; bones soft.
Often have large heads with stomachs like inverted saucers.
Profuse head sweats which soak pillow during sleep.
Can stick their feet out of bed.
Chilly yet get hot on slightest exertion.
Always feel better when constipated.

Calcarea Carbonica can be used in the following complaints providing symptoms agree:

Colds: Takes cold very easily at every change in weather. Nostrils sore, ulcerated. Nose stopped up, also with fetid, yellow discharge. Sneezing. Nose bleeds.

Constipation: Children feel much better when constipated. Stool large at first, then pasty, then liquid. Can be useful in diarrhoea of children.

Ear Troubles: Throbbing, cracking in ears. Pulsating pain pressing outwards. Sensitive to cold about ears and neck.

Headache: Open fontanelles, head enlarged. Much perspiration, wets the pillow. Headache with cold hands and feet. Headache from mental exercise. Head feels hot and heavy with pale face.

Insomnia: Night terrors, they wake up screaming in early hours but remember nothing.

Stomach Troubles: Frequent sour belching. Milk disagrees. Loss of appetite when overworked. Longing for cold drinks. Craving for indigestible things – chalk, coal, pencils!, also for eggs, salt and sweets. Thirst for cold drinks.

Throat Troubles: Large tonsils, cervical glands swollen. Stitches on swallowing. Hawking up mucus. Difficult swallowing. Often have adenoids.

Worms: One of the remedies to be considered for worms.

CALCAREA PHOSPHORICA

The following characteristics are often found in children who need this remedy:

Children are inclined to be thin, pale, lanky, overgrown, with flabby, sunken abdomens, are weak, peevish, fretful and restless, continually wanting change.

Defective nutrition, unable to assimilate calcium.

Memory is weak and they are slow to learn.

Anaemic.

Cold weather and every change of weather brings on ailments.

All ailments are better by rest.

Worse by exertion and in cold weather; worse also by thinking of the pain.

Calcarea Phosphorica can be used in the following complaints providing the symptoms agree:

Diarrhoea: Stools green and spluttering caused by much flatulence. Ice cream, fruit and cold drinks cause diarrhoea.

Headache: Headaches of anaemic school girls and children at puberty, worse from wearing a hat and any jar. Heat of head with smarting at roots of hair. Tendency to head sweats. In early years fontanelles are slow to close.

Extremities: Muscular growing pains. Weak ankles and children are often late in learning to walk. They are unable to assimilate the calcium needed for the formation of strong bones. Helpful in all cases of fracture.

Mouth Troubles: Because they cannot assimilate calcium teeth are slow to erupt and then decay easily. Teething is accompanied by diarrhoea.

Stomach Troubles: Infants wants to nurse all the time and vomit easily. Easy vomiting of children. Colicky pain on attempting to eat.

Throat Troubles: Enlarged glands and tonsils but especially adenoids. Colds settle in throat and every cold brings on tonsillitis.

CAPSICUM

Characteristics:

Fat, red-faced chilly people of lax fibre; clumsy, awkward, unwashed.

Homesickness with red face and sleeplessness.

Burning sensations and burning pains worse cold applications and found in chilly people.

Tendency to inflammatory conditions of ears.

Explosive cough expelling fetid air from lungs and causing bad taste.

Worse open air or draught; cold, damp weather.

Better heat.

The following characteristics are often found in children:

They are fat, lazy, obstinate and clumsy in movement.

They can be forgetful because of inattention.

Often irritable and touchy.

They are rather dull and slow to learn.

These children are utterly miserable away from home and capsicum has helped many children who are homesick at boarding school.

They are often thirsty with acute illnesses but shiver after cold drinks for which they ask.

Capsicum can be given in the following complaints providing symptoms agree:

Cough: Pain in distant parts on coughing, knee, legs, ears etc. Cough explosive expelling pungent, fetid air. Worse warm drinks, cold draughts, anger.

Ear Troubles: Swelling and pain behind ears. Infection of middle ear. Burning and stinging in ears. Tender to touch.

Headache: Bursting headache, worse coughing. Hot face, red cheecks.

Mouth Troubles: Fetid odour.

Stomach Troubles: Much thirst but drinking causes shuddering. Burning.

Throat Troubles: Sore but only when not swallowing. Pain and dryness extending to ears. Back of throat feels hot.

CAUSTICUM

Characteristics:

Hopeless and despondent.
Anxious.
Great weakness, often feels faint.
Sinking of strength with trembling, culminating in local paralysis.
Burning – soreness – rawness (soreness as if parts were raw).
Worse in clear, dry weather, extremes of temperature, winds, draughts.
Better in damp, wet weather, warmth of bed.
Chilly people.

The following characteristics are often found in children who need this remedy:
They are delicate, sensitive and sympathetic, cannot bear to see other people upset or crying.
They can be very clumsy; are late in learning to walk and fall easily.
They do not want to go to bed alone, can be very tearful, but laughter follows.

Causticum can be used in the following complaints providing the symptoms agree:

Colds: Sneezing, dry or fluent cold with nose-bleeds. Chronic colds, thick, yellow or green discharge.

Constipation: Frequent but unsuccessful desire for stool, with pain and straining and redness of face; passed more easily standing up.

Cough: Dry and hollow, sensation as though he cannot cough deeply enough to bring up any mucus. Soreness and rawness in larynx and chest. Cough better by drinking cold water.

Ear Troubles: Ear wax. Feeling of obstruction with offensive discharge. Externally ears are red and burning.

Extremities: Slow in learning to walk. Unsteady, tendancy to fall. Restless legs at night. Cold feet. Disturbing dreams. Talks and laughs in sleep.

Fever: Chilliness and shivering. Heat worse from 6 to 8 p.m. Sweats while walking in open air.

Influenza: Tired, sore, bruised sensation. Soreness in chest when coughing, with involuntary urination (see also Fever).

Insomnia: Wakens at least noise. Starting, tossing about. Disturbing dreams. Talks and laughs in sleep.

Throat Troubles: Sore and raw. Burning pains not worse swallowing. Feels rough, scraped, shooting pains on swallowing. Mucus in throat. Larynx sore and raw, hoarseness of voice, worse morning.

CHAMOMILLA

Characteristics:

Turmoil in temper. Bad effects from bad temper.
Cannot bear pain. Pains out of proportion to illness.
Numbness with pain.
Driven out of bed by pain.
Restless with rage.
Worse heat, open air, at night.
Better warm, wet weather.

The following characteristics are often found in children:
**Extreme restlessness because of pain which they resent and
so they get into a rage and if given a toy will throw it away and
continue to scream. In this state, usually at night, one cheek is
very red and the other pale.**
**The child likes to jog about and if stopped it will hit out or pull
your hair.**
**Child gets tired of playthings quickly and wants something
else.**

*Chamomilla can be used in the following complaints providing
symptoms agree:*

Diarrhoea: Green stool.

Ear Troubles: Acute pain in ear brought on by exposure to cold.
Child does not want to be touched, is very irritable and often
screaming with pain. Chamomilla is marvellous especially if there
is a flush on the cheek on the side of the pain.

Extremities: Feet burning which they often push out of bed to cool.

Insomnia: Drowsiness. Sometimes wailing during sleep. Nightmares.

Mouth Troubles: Gums tender, much worse any heat, better by cold applications. Teething children have very swollen and inflamed gums which are very tender, usually on one side with a very red flush on that side of the face.

Nervous Troubles: Bad temper, nothing pleases. Great restlessness. Intolerance of everything. Effects of excitement often bring on bilious troubles.

CINCHONA OFFICINALIS

Characteristics:

Extreme debility from loss of fluids such as blood, diarrhoea etc., with increasing anaemia and pallor.
Roaring in ears.
Taste bitter; loathes food; desires spices, stimulants etc.
Sweats on least exertion.
Very sensitive to slight touch – dreads this.
Great flatulence with sensation as though abdomen is packed full; not better by wind up or down.
Very sensitive to cold air and liable to take cold.
Short of breath – exhausted individuals.
Pains tearing, cutting, sticking.
Worse slightest touch; loss of vital fluids; at night.
Better hard pressure; warmth.

China can be given in the following complaints providing symptoms agree:

Diarrhoea: Very debilitating diarrhoea, stools acrid, undigested, watery, involuntary, painless, putrid, profuse.

Fainting: From loss of blood.

Fever: Thirst before chill and during sweat. No thirst during chill. Debilitating night sweats.

Haemorrhages: The results of excessive or prolonged bleeding from nose, throat, uterus or any orifice.

GELSEMIUM

Characteristics:

Dizziness, drowsiness, dullness and trembling.
Terrors of anticipation; fearful.
Muscular weakness, langour, listless.
Tiredness – limbs feel tired.

The following characteristics are often found in children:
**Small child dizzy when carried, clutches mother fearing that
he will fall.**
Good remedy for children.

*Gelsemium can be given in the following complaints providing
symptoms agree:*

Colds: Sneezing, fullness at root of nose. Watery, excoriating
discharge, with dull headache and fever.

Diarrhoea: From emotional excitement, anticipation, fear.

Fever: Chilliness, aches all over, does not want to move. Dull
headache, heavy limbs. Chills up and down back. No thirst.

Hay Fever: Violent sneezing, nose streams worse in morning. Eyes
hot and heavy. Much tingling in nose. Throat dry and burning. Face
hot, tired and aching.

Headache: Feeling of band around head, pain at back of head. Dull
heavy ache, eyelids heavy. Pain in temple extending to ear. Nervous headaches. Headaches always better for profuse urination.

Influenza: Typical flu picture, chills run up and down spine, hot and cold. Great heaviness and tiredness of body and limbs especially of head and eyelids. Aches all over. Sneezing; hard cough; bursting headache from back of neck to eyes and forehead.

Measles: Chills and heat chase one another. Fever. Extreme prostration. Sneezing and sore throat, nasal discharge. Severe heavy headache. Drowsy, eyelids heavy; eyes inflamed. No thirst. Gelsemium helps to bring out the rash.

Nervous Troubles: Depression, sometimes after flu. Listless, does not wish to make any effort. Fear of falling, shaky.

HEPAR SULPHURIS

Characteristics:

Hyper sensitive. Irritible. Impetuous. General sensitivity to all impressions, the slightest cause irritates.
Very sensitive to pain.
Feels as if wind is blowing on to some part.
Tendency to suppurations.
Sweats easily on slight exertion.
Better damp weather. Warmth. Wrapped up head. After eating.
Worse dry cold wind. Cool air. Slightest draught.

Hepar Sulph. can be used in the following complaints providing symptoms agree:

Abscess: When pus has formed. Sharp, stabbing pain. Very tender. Worse cold.

Colds: Sneezes every time he goes out into a cold, dry wind, with running nose which later thickens to yellow mucus. Nose stopped up each time he goes out into cold air. Infected sinus with pus forming, will often start the draining of mucus in stuffy colds. Must be well wrapped up.

Coughs: Bouts of dry hoarse coughing, worse cold dry weather and breathing cold air. Worse uncovering any part of the body, even putting hand out of bed. Patient is chilly, sweaty and thirsty for hot drinks.

Croup: Aconite, Spongia, Hepar Sulph. See under Aconite. Hepar Sulph., croup is accompanied with rather loose cough with wheezing and rattling. Worse least breath of cold air. Stitching pains, desires to be warmly wrapped up.

Diarrhoea: Sour smelling, white, clay coloured, green, slimy. Worse during day, after eating and after drinking cold water. Whole child smells sour.

Ear Troubles: Tendency to suppuration, fetid pus. Pain in ear with redness, heat, itching. Worse draught.

Eye Troubles: Chronic and with a tendency to styes.

Fainting: From slight pain.

Skin Troubles: Unhealthy, every little injury suppurates. Sores which fester, sensitive to touch and worse cold air. Sharp pains. Very sensitive cold sores.

Throat Troubles: Sensation of crumb stuck in throat. Pain shoots from throat into ears; throat very sensitive internally and externally. Pain in larynx when swallowing food. Irritable, sensitive to cold draughts.

Toothache: Teeth very sensitive. Gums bleed easily.

IGNATIA

Characteristics:

A remedy of contradictions.
Mental stresses and strains from shock, bereavement, fright etc.
Much grief, long sighs, sobbing, unhappiness.
Twitching, spasms or convulsions from depression, fright, emotions etc.
Great aversion to tobacco smoke.
Weak, empty sensation in stomach not relieved by eating.
Changeable moods. Nash says 'Ignatia may justly be termed pre-eminently the remedy of MOODS.'
Worse slight touch, coffee, smoking.
Better lying on painful side, hard pressure, profuse watery urination.

The following characteristics are often found in children:
This is a highly strung child, bright, sensitive and precocious and when over-worked the nervous system suffers.
Some children will become excited and cry or get depressed, others will look strained and depleted and may find speaking difficult.

Ignatia can be given in the following complaints providing symptoms agree:

Cough: Dry, irritating, spasmodic cough which comes on at inconvenient times. Coughing increases the desire to cough and it goes on and on. Child very stressed. Or an acute dry, spasmodic cough with tendency to spasm of larynx.

Fainting: From excitement.

Headache: Tired, nervous headache coming on at the end of the day after stress. Head congested. Better hot applications.

Nervous Troubles: Caused by shock or strain. Depression and irritability but moods change rapidly.

Stomach Troubles: Digestive upsets by simple food but patient can digest the most indigestible meal. Hiccough after eating, drinking or emotional upset.

Throat Troubles: Acute, inflamed and sore. Tonsils inflamed, swollen with sore ulcers.

LYCOPODIUM

Characteristics:

Apprehension and fears when anticipating an unusual event. Dread of solitude though not wishing for too much company (would like to live alone but know that somebody was in another part of the house).
After eating a few mouthsful feels full up.
All symptoms right-sided or going from right to left.
The 4 p.m. to 8 p.m. aggravation (all symptoms are worse between these times).
Extreme tendency to flatulence with its intolerence to tight clothing.
Worse 4 to 8 p.m. Cold food and drink. Oysters (sick).
Better Open air. Movement. Warm drinks.

The following characteristics are often found in children who need this remedy:
These children are thin and can be sallow.
They are rather diffident and lack assurance, need a lot of support.
Peevish and irritable.
They are liable to digestive upsets but have a very good appetite although they often do not put on weight.
They love sweets, and prefer hot food.
They are chilly but tend to be sensitive to stuffy atmospheres.

Lycopodium can be used in the following complaints providing the symptoms agree:

Colds: Nose stopped up with thick, yellow mucus or yellow or green crusts and a post-nasal drip (dropping down at the back of the throat). Stopped up nose.

Cough: Tickling, deep, hollow. Thick, grey purulent mucus. Tickling night cough.

Headache: Pressing on top of head. Throbbing headache with every spasm of coughing. Pain over eyes in severe colds. Pains worse in a warm room and better exercise in open air but they feel chilly.

Nervous Troubles: Very emotional, easily moved to tears. Nervous, apprehensive when asked to do anything unusual. Irritated quickly.

Stomach Troubles: After eating a little they feel bloated and uncomfortable and are full of wind. This is why they cannot bear anything tight round the waist. Crave sweets and sweet things which make them sick. Worse flatulent foods, e.g. cabbage, beans etc. Milk disagrees and they cannot take cold food or drink.

Throat Troubles: Dryness without thirst. Inflammation with stitches on swallowing. Swelling and suppuration of tonsils. Ulceration of tonsils. Symptoms begin on right side and spread to left. Better warm drinks. Worse cold drinks.

Urination: There is often a red sediment in the urine which tends to improve some symptoms. There is sometimes a delay in starting to urinate, and an increase in urine at night. Child may cry before urinating.

MERCURIUS

Characteristics:

Profuse, fetid sweats which give no relief.
Breath very offensive as are all discharges.
Gums spongy, bleeding.
Tongue flabby and swollen. Takes imprint of teeth.
Profuse salivation.
Creeping chilliness at beginning of disease.
Trembling of limbs.
Rest ameliorates but warmth of bed aggravates.
Worse from both heat and cold and at night.
Always worse lying on right side.

Mercurius can be given in the following complaints providing symptoms agree:

Colds: Sneezing; nostrils raw and ulcerated; nasal bones swollen. Yellow-green fetid pus-like discharge. Sore, raw, smarting sensation, profuse, fluent. Worse in damp weather.

Cough: Worse lying on right side, worse at night. Yellow mucus.

Diarrhoea: Stool greenish, bloody and slimy, worse at night, with pain. Putrid odour.

Ear Troubles: Thick yellow discharge, fetid and bloody. Pains worse at night. Boils in external canal.

Fever: Caused by humid weather. Alternation of chilliness and warmth. Profuse sweat gives no relief. Extreme thirst although mouth moist. Worse at night.

Mouth Troubles: Tongue soft and flabby. Gums spongy and bleed easily. Gumboils. Teeth become loose and gums recede. Breath is foul. Mouth ulcers. Thirst in spite of moist tongue.

Mumps: Especially of right side. Foul tongue. Offensive sweat and salivation.

Skin Troubles: Constantly moist. Great tendency to free perspiration but patient not relieved.

Throat Troubles: Ulcers and inflammation at every change in the weather. Stitches into ear on swallowing. Sore, raw, smarting, burning in throat. Loss of voice.

Whooping Cough: with nose bleed.

NATRUM MURIATICUM

Characteristics:

Ill effects of grief, fright, anger. Worse consolation and fuss.
Cannot weep or weeps in privacy of own room.
Depressed, moody.
Wants solitude.
Lachrymation from laughter and in a wind.
Desires salt. Loathes fat.
Cannot urinate in the presence of others.
Aggravation and amelioration at the seaside.
Worse heat and cold. Sun.
Better open air. Cold bathing.

The following characteristics are often found in children:
These children are often underweight and even when very young prefer to be left alone and dislike being handled, they resent it.
They cry more from rage than fear.
Never try to soothe these children as this makes them worse.
They often knock things over because they do things in a hurry.
Although chilly they are worse heat and cold and cannot stand the sun which always gives them a hammering headache.

Colds: Much sneezing, discharge watery or like the white of an egg which irritates nose. Stopped up nose with loss of smell and taste. Boericke says 'This remedy is infallible for stopping a cold which commences with sneezing.'

Eye Troubles: Feel bruised with headaches of school children. Watering on coughing. Watering in a wind. Watering with laughter.

Headaches: Often pre-menstrual but very common after a long journey, or a visit to the theatre, from eye-strain, mental exertion or excitement. Starts at back and spreads all over the head. Sometimes caused by frontal sinus inflammation. Often throbbing pains like little hammers – can start in the morning. Frontal headaches of school children, working too hard, with pressure over the eyes.

Mouth Troubles: Cold sores around mouth, worse at the seaside. Tingling and numbness of the tongue.

Skin Troubles: Greasy.

Stomach Troubles: Craving for salt, children often steal it. Unquenchable thirst.

Whooping Cough: When there is a flow of tears with cough.

NUX VOMICA

Characteristics:

Irritable, fiery temperament, can get excited, angry, spiteful and malicious.
Easily offended, very sensitive – sullen, fault finding.
Worse morning, mental exertion, over-eating and over-drinking. Dry cold weather; very chilly people cannot get warm.
Better from a nap. Evening. Resting and in damp, wet weather.
A predominantly male remedy.

Nux Vomica can be used in the following complaints providing symptoms agree:

Asthma: Attack often follows a stomach upset with much belching. Patient irritable.

Colds: Stuffy. Snuffles in children worse in warm room. Runny nose in day-time, stuffed up at night and out of doors.

Constipation: With frequent ineffectual urging, feeling as if part remained unexpelled.

Cough: Dry with sore larynx and chest. Sometimes ends in retching. More prevalent in cold, dry, windy weather. Shivers when moving.

Diarrhoea: Caused by excessive food. Alternates with constipation. Worse in morning.

Hay Fever: Great irritation in nose, eyes and face. Long periods of sneezing. Face feels as if close to hot plate.

Headache: At back of head or over the eyes, sometimes with giddiness. Or a frontal headache with desire to press the head against something hard. Intoxicated feeling worse morning, mental exertion, tobacco, alcohol, coffee, open air, better warmth, lying down, warm, moist weather.

Inlfuenza: Cold even in bed, least exposure intensifies cold sensation. Aching limbs and back. Very irritable.

Nervous Troubles: Tense, quarrelsome, critical, very sensitive. Annoyed by little things.

Stomach Troubles: Caused by over-eating. Better sitting or lying down.

At the beginning of many acute conditions the patient needing Nux Vomica will begin to feel cold – this will intensify and no matter how many extra clothes he puts on the coldness remains even when sitting very near a large fire. He is very irritable and will snap at the least thing and very often say he feels sick and would feel better if he could vomit.

PHOSPHORUS

Characteristics:

Mentally active, sensitive, full of fears. Fears thunderstorms and are affected by electrical changes in atmosphere. Fear of being alone, of dark, diseases, death etc. Worse at twilight until midnight.

Affectionate, yet in illness indifferent to loved ones. Desires to be rubbed and mesmerised.

Burning pains better from warmth, heat and hot applications but stomach and head are worse from heat and relieved by cold.

Craves cold drinks, ice cream etc., but as soon as liquids become warm in stomach they are vomited.

Bright, free flowing haemorrhages.

Worse lying on left side.

The following characteristics are often found in children:

A slight and rather delicate child, nervy and excitable, anxious, sensitive, dislikes being alone, is afraid of the dark and thunder. This child is very affectionate, will go into mothers room for affection and returns it.

They are very observant children and will watch everything that goes on around them. Their eyes will follow every movement of the doctor for instance, probably from apprehension. They are warm, outgoing children and would not want to hurt anybody.

They are inclined to flush after excitement or hot food.

Symptoms are apt to strike suddenly – everything comes suddenly, a profuse nose-bleed; a violent temperature etc.

Phosphorus can be used in the following complaints providing symptoms agree:

57

Colds: Go to larynx and chest causing loss of voice. Often one nostril runs and the other is blocked; nose bleeds often. Chest feels tight, burning pains. Chronic catarrh with small nose bleeds, handkerchief is always bloody. Sensitive to smell.

Cough: From tickling in throat, worse cold air, talking, going from warm room into cold air. Hard, dry, tight, hacking cough. Tightness in chest.

Haemorrhage: Bright red, flows freely. Easy bleeding and easy bruising everywhere.

Headaches: Congestive, throbbing, often accompanied by or preceded by hunger but worse from hot food. Worse any kind of heat and by lying down. Better from rest, cold applications and by eating.

Stomach Troubles: Hunger soon after eating. Sour taste. Belching. Water is vomited as soon as it gets warm in the stomach. Stomachache relieved by cold food, ices. Bad effects from eating too much salt.

Wounds: Bleed very much even if small.

PULSATILLA

Characteristics:

Mentally an April day, upset one minute and laughing the next.
Symptoms are always changing.
They love fuss and want affection.
Affectionate.
Can be irritable.
Craving for fresh air and they must have it although they can be chilly.
Cannot bear heat in ANY FORM.
Never thirsty even with a fever.
Worse fat and greasy foods. Rich foods (although nearly all people requiring this remedy eat and enjoy butter!). Heat. Sun. Hot rooms.
Better walking slowly in fresh air.

The following characteristics are often found in children:
A very loving, affectionate, clinging child, rather demanding, wants a lot of attention; shy.
Most Pulsatilla children are afraid of the dark and being left alone.
Changeable rather like an April day of sunshine and showers, laughing one minute and crying the next. Can be irritable.
Hot and sweaty, always flags in the heat but acute conditions are likely to come from being chilled in hot weather or a sudden change from hot to cold weather.
Child is liable to become giddy when looking up at anything high.

Pulsatilla can be given in the following complaints providing symptoms agree:

Colds: Acute colds in the head with nose running; child is shivery and very chilly. Nose is stuffed up indoors and at night but runs in open air. Discharge is bland. Thick creamy, yellow/green catarrh.

Cough: Dry in evening, loose in morning. Gagging and choking, thick yellow mucus. Worse in warm room. Better in open air.

Ear Troubles: Redness and swelling of ear. Pain very intense, usually brought on from exposure to cold, and spreads all over side of face and also into throat. Ear feels stopped up. Sometimes discharge thick, bland, yellowy-green. Worse warmth, evening, night. Better fresh air.

Eyes Troubles: *Conjunctivitis*, eyes very sensitive to cold draughts and water profusely in open air. Eyelids itch. Styes affecting lower lid.

Extremities: Chilblains worse heat.

Fainting: From hot, stuffy atmosphere.

Headaches: Pain in temples and throbbing all over head. Worse in stuffy room, lying down, stooping and in the evening. Better from pressure, walking gently in open air.

Measles: But not when patient has a very high fever. There is catarrh, profuse lachrymation, dry mouth, seldom thirst. Cough that is troublesome. Wants air. Very restless and irritable, wants attention.

Mumps: Lingering fever, and complications which cause swelling in testicles or breasts.

Stomach Troubles: Upsets from rich, fat food. Pain in stomach soon after eating. No thirst. Burning pain. Feels bloated.

Toothache: Great pain. Worse heat and hot fluids. Better cold water. Mouth dry. No thirst.

SILICA

Characteristics:

Lack of grit, moral and physical.
Faint-hearted, anxious, very sensitive.
Adult has fixed ideas.
Always wants head covered and wrapped up warmly.
Offensive odour from feet with or without sweat.
Cold extremities even in a warm room.
Suppuration – Silica expels pus and foreign bodies.
Better warmth.

The following characteristics are often found in children:
Timidity, frightened, yielding, giving up very easily in any difficult situation yet they can be very obstinate and irritable and capable of getting into a rage; they can be so sensitive that even when spoken to kindly they can burst into tears.
They shirk any kind of responsibility because they fear failure.
They are timid, shy and easily embarrassed.
They have definite ideas and are very conscientious. Fairly bright mentally but easily tired out mentally.
Very sensitive to pain and to noise.
Except for a large head and abdomen this child is thin and under nourished; late in starting to walk.
Any exertion causes children to become overheated and they then take cold easily.

Silica can be given in the following complaints providing symptoms agree:

Abscess: Opens them to expel pus. Will expel foreign bodies, splinters etc.

Colds: Dry, hard crusts form in nose, bleeding when loosened. Sneezing. Obstructed and loss of smell.

Constipation: Common in children needing silica – they have a 'bashful' stool which is partially expelled with much straining only to slip back.

Cough: Colds do not yield, cough develops. Violent when lying down with thick, yellow, lumpy expectoration.

Extremities: Foot sweat very offensive – feet can exude a terrible odour even without sweat. This sweat should never be suppressed as many chronic ailments can result. Silica can restore the sweating and then the child can be cured. Crippled nails.

Headache: Pain starts in nape of neck and comes up over top of head and settles in one eye; usually the right. Pressure of hat makes pain worse yet patient wants head wrapped up and kept warm. Head feels cold and every draught of air is felt. Head sweats profusely.

Skin Troubles: Abscesses, boils, ulcers. Every little injury suppurates.

Stomach Troubles: Craves ice cream, cold food and cold drinks – there is a definite dislike of hot food. Poor assimilation of food, especially milk which accounts for poor physique (soft bones, poor nails, poor teeth which decay readily at the margins).

Throat Troubles: Colds settle in throat. Pricking in tonsil; stinging pains on swallowing. Glands swollen.

SULPHUR

Characteristics:

Selfish people – rather lazy.
Untidy, fling themselves into a chair.
Philosophical, want to know why and wherefore of things.
Skin burning and itching.
Red orifices – eyes, nose, ears, anus.
Sinking feeling mid-morning, poor breakfast eaters.
Offensive discharges – acrid and excoriating making part over which they flow red and burning.
Worse warmth of bed, great heat, morning, standing.
Better dry, warm weather.

The following characteristics are often found in children:
They can be boastful about their belongings.
They can show intense curiosity about everything, wanting to know how things work etc.
Can be irritable and quarrelsome.
Some tend to be lazy.

Sulphur can be given in the following complaints providing symptoms agree:

Colds: Dry scabs; and bleeding from nose.

Constipation: Hard stools, child afraid on account of pain.

Cough: Loose with greenish, purulent, sweetish expectoration; there is much rattling of mucus. Worse talking, morning.

Diarrhoea: Habitual early morning stool driving child out of bed because of urgency. Diarrhoea painless. Redness around anus.

Extremities: Hands often hot and sweaty. Burning in soles and hands at night; feet often put out of bed to cool.

Eye Troubles: Burning in eyes. Burning and redness of lids.

Headache: Heat on top of head. Sick headache recurring periodically. Heaviness and fullness. Beating headache worse stooping. Scalp dry and itching.

Mouth Troubles: Lips dry – bright red and burning.

Stomach Troubles: Great desire for sweets; milk disagrees. Can be weak and faint about 11 a.m.

REPERTORY OF CHARACTERISTIC SYMPTOMS

Mind Symptoms

Affectionate: *Phos., Puls.*
All symptoms worse after exposure to dry cold winds: *Acon.*
Anger: *Nat.m., Nux.v.*
Anxiety: *Acon., Arg.n., Ars.alb., Caust., Lyc., Phos., Sil.*
Apprehension: *Arg.n., Gels., Lyc.*
Cannot bear to be looked at: *Ant.c.*
Claustrophobic: *Arg.n.*
Debility: *Ant.t., China., Gels.*
Depressed: *Bar.c., Ign., Nat.m.*
Despondent: *Caust.*
Dreads Strangers: *Bar.c.*
Drowsiness: *Ant.t., Gels.*
Dullness: *Gels.*
Easily upset: *Ant.c.*
Exciteable: *Bell., Phos.*
Fastidious: *Ars.alb.*
Fault finding: *Nux.v.*
Fearful: *Acon., Arg.n., Ars.alb., Calc.c., Gels., Lyc., Phos.*
Funks examinations: *Arg.n.*
Homesick: *Caps.*
Impulsive: *Arg.n., Hep.s.*
Irrational thoughts: *Arg.n.*
Irresolute: *Bar.c.*
Irritable: *Ant.t., Bry., Calc.p., Caps., Hep.s., Nux.v., Puls.*
Lacks grit: *Sil.*
Lazy: *Sulph.*
Malicious: *Nux.v.*
Memory deficient: *Bar.c.*
Memory weak: *Calc.p.*

Moods changing: *Ign.*, *Nat.m.*
Obstinate: *Caps.*, *Sil.*
Peevish: *Ant.c.*, *Calc.p.*
Philosophical: *Sulph.*
Prostration: *Ars.alb.*
Restless: *Ars.alb.*, *Bell.*, *Calc.p.*, *Cham.*
Selfish: *Sulph.*
Sensitive: *Ant.c.*, *Caust.*, *China.*, *Hep.s.*, *Nux.v.*, *Phos.*, *Sil.*
Solitude, desires: *Nat.m.*
Tearful: *Caust.*
Temper: *Cham.*
Tension: *Acon.*
Timid: *Bar.c.*, *Sil.*
Tiredness: *Gels.*
Untidy: *Sulph.*
Weakness: *Ant.t.*, *Caust.*
Worse consolation and fuss: *Nat.m.*
Worse heights: *Arg.n.*
Worse fright: *Nat.m.*

GENERAL CHARACTERISTICS

Acute, sudden, violent invasion with fever: *Acon.*
Aversion tobacco smoke: *Ign.*
Breathless: *Calc.c.*
Child does not want pulse taken: *Ant.t.*
Child wants to be carried but cries if touched: *Ant.t.*
Child clumsy: *Ant.c.*
Child fair, fat, chilly, lethargic and sweaty: *Calc.c.*
Child highly strung: *Ign.*
Child physically undersize: *Bar.c.*
Child with low stamina: *Calc.c.*
Chilliness at beginning of disease: *Merc.*
Chilly but hot on slightest exertion: *Calc.c.*
Chilly, needs much clothing: *Bar.c.*
Cold extremities even in warm room: *Sil.*
Complaints develop slowly: *Bry.*
Craves cold drinks: *Phos.*
Craves eggs: *Calc.c.*
Craves fresh air: *Puls.*
Craves ice-cream: *Phos.*
Craves indigestible things: *Calc.c.*
Debility extreme from loss of fluids: *China.*
Desires salt: *Nat.m.*
Desires sugar which makes him worse: *Arg.n.*
Desires sweet things: *Arg.n., Lyc., Sulph.*
Derangements from overloading stomach: *Ant.c.*
Eating a few mouthsful gives full feeling: *Lyc.*
Faintness sitting up in bed: *Bry.*
Feet feel as if wearing cold, damp stockings: *Calc.c.*
Fever with hot, dry, burning skin: *Bell.*
Feverish conditions at night: *Ant.c.*
Fingernails grow in splits with horny spots: *Ant.c.*
Flabby: *Calc.c.*

Flatulence: *China., Lyc.*
Haemorrhages: *Phos.*
Hand soft, cool, boneless: *Calc.c.*
Head always wants to be wrapped up warmly: *Sil.*
Homesickness: *Caps.*
Intolerance of tight clothing: *Lyc.*
Lachrymation with laughter: *Nat.m.*
Lachrymation in wind: *Nat.m.*
Liquids vomited as soon as warm in stomach: *Phos.*
Loathes fat: *Nat.m., Puls.*
Mucus accumulation with much rattling and inability to raise: *Ant.t.*
Mucus, dryness of membranes: *Bry.*
Muscular weakness: *Gels.*
Offensive breath and all discharges: *Merc.*
Offensive odour from feet with or without sweat: *Sil.*
Offensive discharges: *Sulph.*
Orifices red: *Sulph.*
Pains – burning: *Caust., Sulph.*
        burning better heat but wants head cool: *Ars.alb.*
        burning worse cold applications: *Caps.*
        burning better warmth, heat and hot applications: *Phos.*
        cannot bear: *Cham.*
        cutting: *China.*
        motion, worse: *Bry.*
        numbness, with: *Cham.*
        rawness: *Caust.*
        Sensitive to: *Hep.s.*
        Soreness: *Caust.*
        Stabbing: *Bry.*
        Sticking: *China.*
        Stitching: *Bry.*
        Tearing: *China.*
        Throbbing: *Bell.*
Pupils dilated: *Bell.*
Sensitive to cold air: *China.*
Sinking feeling mid-morning: *Sulph.*
Skin burning: *Sulph.*
Skin hot: *Acon.*
Skin dry: *Acon.*

Skin itching: *Sulph.*
Slow in cutting teeth: *Calc.c.*
Slow in walking: *Calc.c.*
Slowness: *Calc.c.*
Sudden beginning of any illness with fever, anxiety, restlessness
   and fear: *Acon.*
Sudden rise in temperature: *Bell.*
Suppuration: *Hep.s., Sil.*
Sweats easily on slight exertion: *Hep.s.*
Sweat profuse, cold about head: *Calc.c.*
             fetid with no relief: *Merc.*
             on head which soaks the pillow: *Calc.c.*
Sweats on slight exertion: *China.*
Symptoms right sided or going from right to left: *Lyc.*
Thirst for copious draughts at long intervals: *Bry.*
Thirst lack of: *Ant.c.*
Thirst never even with fever: *Puls.*
Tiredness: *Gels.*
Tongue thickly coated, very white: *Ant.c.*
Tongue flabby and swollen: *Merc.*
Urinate, cannot in the presence of others: *Nat.m.*
Weak, empty feeling in stomach not better by eating: *Ign.*
Weakness, often feels faint: *Caust.*
Wind, as if blowing on part of body: *Hep.s.*

MODALITIES

Better: ... Breakfast, after: *Calc.c.*
Cold air: *Arg.n.*
Cold bathing: *Nat.m.*
Cold things: *Bry.*
Constipated, when: *Calc.c.*
Dark, in the: *Calc.c.*
Drawing up limbs: *Calc.c.*
Eating, after: *Hep.s.*
Evening: *Nux.v.*
Expectoration: *Ant.t.*
Garments, loosening: *Calc.c.*
Lying on back: *Calc.c.*
Lying on painful side: *Bry., Ign.*
Movement: *Lyc.*
Nap, having a: *Nux.v.*
Pressure: *Bry.*
Pressure, hard: *Chin., Ign.*
Rest: *Bry., Calc.p., Merc., Nux.v.*
Rubbing: *Calc.c.*
Sitting erect: *Ant.t.*
Urination, profuse, watery: *Ign.*
Warm drinks: *Lyc.*
Warmth: *Ars.alb., Caps., China., Hep.s., Sil.*
Warmth of bed: *Caust.*
Wind, bringing up: *Ant.t.*
Wrapping up head: *Hep.S. Sil.*

Air, open: *Acon., Lyc., Nat.m.*
Damp weather: *Hep.s.*
Damp, wet weather: *Caust., Nux.v.*
Dry, warm weather: *Calc.c., Sulph.*
Walking slowly in fresh air: *Puls.*
Warm, wet weather: *Cham.*

MODALITIES

Worse: ... Bathing: *Calc.c.*
Coffee: *Ign.*
Cold applications: *Ars.àlb.*
    bathing: *Ant.c.*
    drinks: *Ars.alb., Lyc.*
    food: *Lyc.*
Consolation and fuss: *Nat.m.*
Draughts: *Caps., Caust., Hep.s.*
Eating, after: *Bar.c.*
Exertion: *Calc.p.*
Fat and greasy foods: *Puls.*
Heat: *Ant.t., Arg.n., Cham., Puls., Sulph.*
Heat of sun: *Ant.c., Puls.*
Hot rooms: *Puls.*
Letting limbs hang down: *Calc.c.*
Loss of vital fluids: *China.*
Lying down at night: *Ant.t.*
    on left side: *Phos.*
    on right side: *Merc.*
Mental exertion: *Nux.v.*
Mental and physical exertion: *Calc.c.*
Morning: *Calc.c.*
Motion, slightest: *Bry*
Over-eating: *Nux.v.*
Pressure of clothes: *Calc.c.*
Radiated heat: *Ant.c.*
Seaside: *Nat.m.*
Smoking: *Ign.*
Standing: *Sulph.*
Stooping: *Calc.c.*
Touch, slightest: *China., Ign.*
Waking, on: *Calc.c.*

Water, working in: *Calc.c.*
Warm room: *Acon., Arg.n., Puls.*
Warmth of bed: *Merc., Sulph.*

Air, open: *Calc.c., Caps., Cham.*
Air, cold: *Ars.alb., Calc.c.*
Clear, dry weather: *Caust.*
Cold weather: *Calc.p.*
Damp weather: *Bry.*
Damp, cold weather: *Ant.t., Calc.c., Caps.*
Dry, cold weather: *Nux.v.*
Dry cold winds: *Acon., Hep.s.*
Extremes of temperature: *Caust.*
Heat and cold: *Merc., Nat.m.*
Sun: *Nat.m.*
Warm weather: *Ant.c.*
Wet weather: *Ars.alb.*
Winds: *Caust.*

4–8 p.m.: *Lyc.*
Evening: *Ant.c.*
Night: *Cham., China., Merc.*
Around mid-night: *Acon.*
After midnight: *Calc.c.*
1–3 a.m.: Ars.alb.
Morning: *Nux.v., Sulph.*

Full moon: *Calc.c.*
New moon: *Calc.c.*

GENERAL REPERTORY

Abscess
Pain: Burning: *Ars.alb., Bell.*
> Burning, better heat: *Ars.alb.*
> Sharp: *Hep.s.*
> Stabbing: *Ars.alb., Hep.s.*
> Throbbing: *Bell.*

Pus, opens to expel: *Sil.*
Pus, when formed: *Hep.s.*
Restless: *Ars.alb.*
Swelling, bright red: *Bell.*
Tender: *Hep.s.*
Worse: after midnight: *Ars.alb.*
> Cold: *Hep.s.*

Asthma
Attack often follows stomach upset with much belching: *Nux.v.*
Breath, shortness of: *Ant.t.*
Breathing difficult: *Ant.t., Ars.alb.*
Breathing difficult worse 1–2 a.m.: *Ars.alb.*
Cannot lie down: *Ars.alb.*
Desires to sit up: *Ant.t.*
Mucus full of, but none comes up: *Ant.t.*
With burning in chest: *Ars.alb.*
With great debility: *Ars.alb.*
Worse: Cold air: *Ars.alb.*
> Motion: *Ars.alb.*
> Better: Bending forward: *Ars.alb.*
> > Heat, applied: *Ars.alb.*
> > Hot drinks: *Ars.alb.*

Chicken-Pox
Bronchitis, often with: *Ant.t.*

Drowsy: *Ant.t.*
Early stages: *Ant.t.*
Eruptions come out slowly: *Ant.t.*
Face flushed: *Bell.*
Headache severe: *Bell.*
Initial stages: *Acon.*
Initial stages with anxiety and restlessness: *Acon.*
Nausea: *Ant.t.*
Peevish: likes company: *Ant.t.*
Skin very hot: *Bell.*
Sweats freely: *Ant.t.*

Colds
After becoming chilled: *Bar.c.*
Chronic: *Caust.*
Eyes red: *Bry.*
Eyes watery: *Bry.*
First sneeze or shiver after exposure to dry cold: *Acon.*
First stage of initial fever with anxiety: *Acon.*
Lip, upper swollen: *Bar.c.*
Mucus Bland: *Puls.*
      Creamy: *Puls.*
      Excoriating: *Gels.*
      Fetid: *Calc.c., Merc.*
      Green: *Caust., Merc., Puls.*
      Little: *Bell.*
      Tenacious: *Acon.*
      Thin, whitish, excoriating: *Ars.alb.*
      Thick: *Acon., Caust., Lyc., Puls.*
      Watery: *Bry., Gels., Nat.m.*
      Whitish pus with clots of blood: *Acon.*
      Yellow: *Calc.c., Caust., Hep.s., Lyc., Merc., Puls.*
Nose: bleeds: *Calc.c., Caust., Phos., Sulph.*
      dry: *Caust.*
      fullness at root of: *Gels.*
      hot: *Bell.*
      itching: *Acon.*
      one nostril blocked the other runs: *Phos.*
      post nasal drip: *Lyc.*
      raw: *Merc.*

Nose: red: *Bell.*
     running: *Bar.c., Bry., Gels., Hep.s.*
     running: daytime: *Nux.v., Puls.*
     running: open air: *Puls.*
     sore: *Bell., Calc.c.*
     stopped up: *Ars.alb., Calc.c., Lyc., Nat.m.*
     stopped up: in cold air: *Hep.s., Sil.*
     stuffy at night: *Nux.v., Puls.*
     stuffy out of doors: *Nux.v.*
     stuffy indoors: *Puls.*
Nose: ulcerated: *Calc.c., Merc.*
Sinus infected: *Hep.s.*
Sneezing frequent: *Acon., Bry., Calc.c., Caust., Gels., Hep.s., Merc., Nat.m., Sil.*
Sneezing frequent without relief: *Ars.alb.*
Symptoms slow to develop: *Bry.*
Takes cold easily: *Bar.c., Calc.c.*
Travels to chest: *Bry., Phos.*
Travels to larynx: *Phos.*
Violent onset: *Bell.*
Worse: Stuffy atmosphere: *Acon., Puls.*
Worse: from midnight to 2 a.m.: *Ars.alb.*

Constipation

Children feel better when constipated: *Calc.c.*
Lips dry: *Bry.*
Mouth dry: *Bry.*
Stools as if burnt: *Bry.*
     dry: *Bry.*
     hard: *Bry., Sulph.*
     large then pasty then liquid: *Calc.c.*
     recedes: *Sil.*
     unsuccessful desire for: *Caust.*
     unsuccessful desire for with pain: *Caust.*
     unsuccessful desire for with straining: *Caust.*
Thirst: *Bry.*
Tongue dry: *Bry.*

Cough

After exposure to dry cold: *Acon.*
Bouts of dry, hoarse coughing: *Hep.s.*
Chronic with swollen glands: *Bar.c.*
Chronic with enlarged tonsils: *Bar.c.*
Compels patient to sit up: *Ant.t.*
Coughing increases desire to cough: *Ign.*
Deep: *Lyc.*
Dry: *Acon., Bell., Bry., Caust., Ign., Nux.v., Puls.*
Dry: evenings: *Puls.*
Explosive: *Caps.*
Hacking: *Phos.*
Hard: *Phos.*
Hollow: *Caust., Lyc.*
Irritating: *Ign.*
Loose with expectoration: *Ant.t.*
Loose mornings: *Puls.*
Pain in distant parts on coughing: *Caps.*
Paroxysms violent: *Bell.*
Retching, sometimes ends in: *Nux.v.*
Short: *Acon.*
Spasmodic: *Bar.c., Ign.*
Tickling: *Bell., Lyc., Phos.*
Tight: *Phos.*
Violent when lying down: *Sil.*
Wakens child from sleep: *Acon.*
With anxiety: *Ars.alb.*
With restlessness: *Ars.alb.*

Chest: Full of mucus: *Bar.c.*
       Pain in: *Ant.t.*
       Rawness: *Caust.*
       Soreness: *Caust.*
       Stitching: *Bry.*
       Tightness: *Phos.*

Head: Bursting feeling: *Bell.*

Larynx: Dryness: *Bell.*
        Pain in: *Ant.t.*

Mucus: Difficult to expel but much there: *Ant.t.*
       Frothy: *Merc., Puls., Sil.*
       Grey: *Lyc.*
       Purulent: *Lyc.*
       Thick: *Lyc., Puls., Sil.*
       Yellow: *Merc., Puls., Sil.*

Respiration: Difficult: *Ars.alb.*
          Wheezing: *Ars.alb.*

Better: Air, open: *Puls.*
     Drinking cold water: *Caust.*

Worse: Anger: *Caps.*
     Breathing cold air: *Hep.s.*
     Cold draughts: *Caps.*
     Cold, dry weather: *Hep.s.*
     Cold, after slightest: *Bar.c.*
     Exposure to dry cold: *Acon.*
     Lying on right side: *Merc.*
     Movement: *Bry.*
     Talking: *Phos.*
     Warm drinks: *Caps.*
     Warm room: *Puls.*
     Warm room on entering: *Acon., Ant.c., Bry.*
     Warm room going from into cold air: *Phos.*

Worse: Uncovering any parts of body: *Hep.s.*
     Evening until midnight: *Bar.c.*
     Midnight until 2 a.m.: *Ars.alb.*
     Night: *Bar.c., Bell., Merc.*

Croup
Accompanied with loose cough: *Hep.s.*
Accompanied with wheezing: *Hep.s.*
Accompanied with rattling: *Hep.s.*

Advanced stages: *Ant.t.*
Chest, difficulty in expanding: *Ant.t.*
Cough loose: *Sulph.*
Expectoration greenish: *Sulph.*
Expectoration purulent: *Sulph.*
Face bluish: *Ant.t.*
Face with cold sweat: *Ant.t.*
Mucus, cannot dislodge: *Ant.t.*
Mucus, rattling: *Sulph.*
Respiration difficult: *Ant.t.*
       shrill: *Ant.t.*
       whistling: *Ant.t.*
Worse least breath of cold air: *Hep.s.*
Better warmly wrapped up: *Hep.s.*

Dandruff
Dry scurf: *Ars.alb.*

Diarrhoea
Alternates with constipation: *Nux.v.*

Causes: Anticipation: *Gels.*
      Cold dry wind: *Acon.*
      Cold drinks: *Calc.p.*
      Drinking cold water when overheated: *Bry.*
      Emotional excitement: *Gels.*
      Excessive food: *Nux.v.*
      Fear: *Gels.*
      Fright: *Acon.*
      Fruit: *Calc.p.*
      Ice-cream: *Calc.p.*
      Sour fruit: *Bry.*

Redness round anus: *Sulph.*

Stool: Acrid: *China.*
     Bloody: *Merc.*
     Clay-coloured: *Hep.s.*
     Debilitating: *China.*
     Green: *Arg.n.*, *Calc.p.*, *Cham.*, *Hep.s.*, *Merc.*
     Involuntary: *China.*

Stool: Painless: *China., Sulph.*
   Profuse: *China.*
   Putrid: *China., Merc.*
   Slimy: *Hep.s., Merc.*
   Sour: *Hep.s.*
   Sour and child smells sour: *Hep.s.*
   Undigested: *China.*
   Watery: *Acon., China.*
   White: *Hep.s.*
   With much flatus: *Arg.n.*

Worse: After drinking cold water: *Hep.s.*
   After eating: *Hep.s.*
   After midnight: *Arg.n.*
   After sweet things: *Arg.n.*
   During the day: *Hep.s.*
   Early morning (stool drives child out of bed): *Sulph.*
   Heat of sun: *Ant.c.*
   Morning: *Nux.v.*
   Night: *Arg.n., Merc.*
   Summer heat: *Ant.c.*

Ear Troubles
Boils in external canal: *Merc.*
From exposure to cold: *Cham., Puls.*

Earache: After chills: *Acon.*
   After exposure to cold: *Acon.*
   Cracking in ear: *Calc.c.*
   Sudden: *Acon., Bell.*

Discharge: Bland: *Puls.*
   Bloody: *Merc.*
   Fetid pus: *Hep.s., Merc.*
   Greenish: *Merc.*
   Offensive: *Caust.*
   Slimy: *Merc.*
   Thick: *Puls.*
   Yellowy-Green: *Merc., Puls.*

Pain: Acute: *Cham.*
      Burning: *Bell., Caps., Caust.*
      Digging: *Bell.*
      Intense: *Puls.*
      Obstruction, feeling of: *Caust., Puls.*
      Pressing outward: *Calc.c.*
      Pulsating: *Calc.c.*
      Stinging: *Caps.*
      Throbbing: *Bell., Calc.c.*
      With heat: *Hep.s.*
      With Itching: *Hep.s.*
      With redness: *Hep.s.*
      Behind ear: *Caps.*
      Worse night: *Merc.*

Redness: *Acon., Caust., Puls.*
Suppuration, tendency to: *Hep.s.*
Swelling: *Puls.*
Swelling behind ear: *Caps.*
Tender to touch: *Caps.*

Better: Fresh air: *Puls.*
       Heat: *Bell.*

Worse: Cold round ears: *Calc.c.*
       Evening: *Puls.*
       Least jar: *Bell.*
       Night: *Puls.*
       Warmth: *Puls.*
       Wax: *Caust.*

Excitement
With fear: *Acon., Bell.*
With headache: *Bell.*
With restlessness: *Acon.*

Extremities
Burning feet: *Cham.*

Burning hands at night: *Sulph.*
Burning soles at night: *Sulph.*
Cold feet: *Caust.*
Fractures: *Calc.p.*
Nails crippled: *Sil.*
Pains, muscular (growing): *Calc.p.*
Restless legs, night: *Caust.*
Sweat, foot: *Sil.*
Sweat, foot offensive: *Sil.*
Unsteady, tendency to fall: *Caust.*
Walking, children late in learning to: *Calc.p., Caust.*
Weak ankles: *Calc.p.*

Eye Troubles
Eyes: Bruised feeling: *Nat.m.*
Burning: *Sulph.*
Burning and redness of lids: *Sulph.*
Itching eyelids: *Puls.*
Sensitive to cold draughts: *Puls.*
Styes affecting lower lids: *Puls.*
Styes chronic: *Hep.s.*
Styes tendency to: *Hep.s.*
Watering on coughing: *Nat.m.*
Watering with laughter: *Nat.m.*
Watering profusely in open air: *Puls.*
Watering in wind: *Nat.m.*

Fainting
From: Atmosphere hot, stuffy: *Puls.*
Blood, loss of: *China.*
Excitement: *Ign.*
Pain, even slight: *Hep.s.*

Fever
Aching: *Gels.*
Agitation: *Acon.*
Alternately hot and cold: *Ars.alb., Barc.c., Merc.*

Alternately hot and cold evening: and night: *Bar.c.*
Chill and chilliness better external warmth: *Bar.c.*
Chills up and down back: *Gels.*
Chilliness: *Caust.*, *Gels.*
Face red: *Acon.*, *Bell.*
Fearful: *Ars.alb.*
Heat worse 6–8 p.m.: *Caust.*
Humid weather, during: *Merc.*
Limbs heavy: *Gels.*
Onset sudden: *Acon.*, *Bell.*
Pains burning, better warmth: *Ars.alb.*
Restless: *Acon.*, *Ars.alb.*
Skin burning: *Acon.*, *Bell.*
Skin dry: *Acon.*
Sweating general: *Bell.*
      at night, debilitating: *Bar.c.*, *China.*
      profuse with no relief: *Merc.*
      walking in open air: *Caust.*
Thirst before chill and during sweat: *China.*
      Great thirst: *Acon.*, *Ars.alb.*
      Great thirst although mouth dry: *Merc.*
      Little: *Bell.*
      None: *Gels.*
Worse after midsnight: *Ars.alb.*
      around midnight: *Acon.*
      evening: *Acon.*
      night: *Merc.*

Haemorrhage
Bleeding excessively or prolonged from nose: *China.*
      excessively or prolonged from throat: *China.*
      excessively or prolonged from uterus: *China.*
Blood flows freely: *Phos.*
Blood bright red: *Phos.*
Bruising easily: *Phos.*

Hay Fever
Discharge profuse: *Ars.alb.*

83

Discharge watery: *Ars.alb.*
Discharge burning: *Ars.alb.*
Eyes burning: *Ars.alb.*
      heavy: *Gels.*
      hot: *Gels.*
      irritation: *Nux.v.*
Face aching: *Gels.*
      hot: *Gels.*, *Nux.v.*
      irritation: *Nux.v.*
Nose Irritation: *Nux.v.*
Nose streams, worse mornings: *Gels.*
      tickles inside: *Ars.alb.*
      tingling: *Gels.*
Restlessness: *Acon.*, *Ars.alb.*, *Bell.*
Sneezing long periods: *Nux.v.*
Sneezing violent: *Ars.alb.*, *Gels.*
Throat burning: *Gels.*
Throat dry: *Gels.*

Headaches
Band, as if tight round head: *Acon.*, *Gels.*
Caused by: Excitement: *Nat.m.*
              Eyestrain: *Nat.m.*
              Long journey; *Nat.m.*
              Mental exercise: *Calc.c.*
              Mental exertion: *Nat.m.*
              Nerves: *Gels.*, *Ign.*
              Pre-menstrual: *Nat.m.*
              Visit to theatre: *Nat.m.*
Chilly, feels: *Lyc.*
Cold head: *Sil.*
Cold head wants it wrapped up: *Sil.*
Enlarged, feels: *Arg.n.*
Fullness: *Sulph.*
Heat on top of head: *Sulph.*
Heat with smarting at roots of hair: *Calc.p.*
Heaviness: *Sulph.*, *Calc.c.*
Heaviness eyelids: *Gels.*
Hot: *Calc.c.*
Intoxicated feeling worse alcohol: *Nux.v.*

84

Intoxicated feeling worse coffee: *Nux.v.*

                   worse mental exertion: *Nux.v.*

                   worse morning: *Nux.v.*

                   worse open air: *Nux.v.*

                   worse tobacco: *Nux.v.*

Of anaemic school-girls: *Calc.p.*

Of anaemic children at puberty: *Calc.p.*

Pains Aching: *Gels.*

Pains Beating worse stooping: *Sulph.*

Pain Bursting: *Bell., Bry., Caps., Gels.*

    Ceases abruptly: *Bell.*

    Pressing: *Arg.n., Lyc.*

    Splitting: *Bry.*

    Sudden: *Acon., Bell.*

    Throbbing: *Bell., Acon., Lyc., Nat.m., Phos., Puls.*

     Throbbing violent: *Bell.*

     in temples: *Puls.*

     in temples extending to ear: *Gels.*

    Eyes over: *Lyx., Nux.v.*

    Forehead: *Bell., Bry.*

    Frontal: *Nat.m., Nux.v.*

    Head, back of: *Gels., Nux.v.*

    Nape of neck over top, settles in one eye: *Sil.*

    Nape of neck spreads all over: *Nat.m.*

    Temples: *Puls.*

    Temples extending to ear: *Gels.*

Scalp dry: *Sulph.*

Scalp Itching: *Sulph.*

Scurf dry: *Bar.c.*

Sensitive to cold: *Bar.c.*

Sick headache: *Sulph.*

Sweating head: *Calc.p., Calc.c., Sil.*

With anxiety: *Acon.*

    Cold hands and feet: *Calc.c.*

    Restlessness: *Acon., Ars.alb.*

    Thirst: *Acon.*

Better: Bending head back: *Bell.*

    Binding head lightly: *Arg.n.*

    Cold air: *Ars.alb.*

Better: Cold applications: *Ars.alb.*, *Phos.*
      Eating: *Phos.*
      Exercise in open air: *Lyc.*
      Hot applications: *Ign.*
      Lying down: *Bell.*, *Nux.v.*, *Phos.*, *Puls.*
      Pressure: *Bell.*, *Puls.*
      Profuse urination: *Gels.*
      Rest: *Phos.*
      Sitting up: *Bell.*
      Walking gently in open air: *Puls.*
      Warmth: *Nux.v.*
      Warm, moist weather: *Nux.v.*

Worse: Evening: *Puls.*
      Heat: *Phos.*
      Jar, any: *Bell.*, *Calc.p.*
      Mental effort: *Arg.n.*
      Motion: *Bry.*
      Movement, violent: *Arg.n.*
      Pressure: *Sil.*
      Stooping: *Puls.*
      Stuffy room: *Puls.*
      Warm room: *Lyc.*
      Wearing a hat: *Calc.p.*

Influenza

Aching limbs: *Bry.*, *Gels.*, *Nux.v.*
Chilliness: *Ars.alb.*
Cold, even in bed: *Nux.v.*
Cold, least exposure intensified: *Nux.v.*
Cough painful: *Bry.*
Heaviness: *Gels.*
Hot and cold chills up and down spine: *Gels.*
Irritable, very: *Nux.v.*
Mental restlessness extreme: *Ars.alb.*
Mental distress: *Ars.alb.*
Pain: Bruised: *Caust.*
      Sore: *Caust.*
      Chest: *Bry.*

Pain: Throat: *Bry.*
Prostration great: *Ars.alb.*
Streaming eyes: *Ars.alb.*
Streaming nose: *Ars.alb.*
Sudden onset: *Acon.*
Sudden onset with chilliness: *Acon.*
           with restlessness: *Acon.*
           with anxiety: *Acon.*
Thirst with dry lips and mouth: *Bry.*
Tiredness of limbs, head and eyelids: *Gels.*
Worse movement: *Bry.*

Insomnia
After midnight: *Ars.alb.*
Awake from fear: *Acon.*
     from fright: *Acon.*
     from least noise: *Caust.*
     from panic: *Acon.*
     from shock: *Acon.*
     screaming from anxious dreams: *Bry.*
     screaming in early hours: *Calc.c.*
Dreams disturbing: *Caust.*
Drowsiness: *Cham.*
Laughs in sleep: *Caust.*
Nightmares: *Cham.*
Night terrors: *Ars.alb., Calc.c.*
Restless: *Acon., Ars.alb.*
Talks in sleep: *Caust.*
Tossing: *Caust.*
Walking during sleep: *Cham.*

Measles
Air desires: *Puls.*
Anxious: *Acon.*
Attention, desires: *Puls.*
Catarrh before rash appears: *Acon.*
Chills and heat alternately: *Gels.*
Cough: *Puls.*
     barking: *Acon.*
     through chest involvement: *Bry.*

Drowsy: *Gels.*
Eyelids heavy: *Gels.*
Eyes inflamed: *Acon., Gels.*
Feet cold but wants air: *Bry.*
Fever: *Gels.*
Fever before rash appears: *Acon.*
Frightened: *Acon.*
Headache severe: *Bry., Gels.*
Irritable: *Puls.*
Lachrymation profuse: *Puls.*
Mouth dry: *Puls.*
Nasal discharge: *Gels., Puls.*
Prostration: *Gels.*
Restless: *Acon., Puls.*
Skin burning: *Acon.*
Skin itching: *Acon.*
Sneezing: *Gels.*
Throat sore: *Gels.*
Thirst nil: *Gels.*
Thirst seldom: *Puls.*

Mouth Troubles

Breath foul: *Merc.*
Gumboils: *Merc.*
Gums bleed easily: *Merc.*
      inflamed: *Cham.*
      recede: *Merc.*
      spongy: *Merc.*
      swollen: *Cham.*
      tender (worse heat better cold applications): *Cham.*
Lips dry: *Sulph.*
    bright red: *Sulph.*
    burning: *Sulph.*
Mouth ulcers: *Merc.*
Odour fetid: *Caps.*
Teeth decay easily: *Calc.p.*
Teeth slow to erupt: *Calc.p.*
Teething children: *Cham.*
Thirst, in spite of moist tongue: *Merc.*

Mumps

Anxiety: *Acon.*
Complications causing swelling in testes: *Puls.*
Complications causing swelling in breasts: *Puls.*
Face glowing red: *Bell.*
Fever lingering: *Puls.*
Inflammation right parotid gland: *Bell.*
Inflammation with bright redness: *Bell.*
Pains shooting: *Bell.*
Pains violent: *Bell.*
Restlessness: *Acon.*
Salivation offensive: *Merc.*
Sweat offensive: *Merc.*
Tongue foul: *Merc.*
Worse right side: *Merc.*

Nervous Troubles

Annoyed about little things: *Nux.v.*
Anxiety before an ordeal: *Arg.n.*, *Gels.*, *Lyc.*
Anxiety extreme: *Acon.*
Apprehension: *Arg.n.*, *Gels.*, *Lyc.*
Claustrophobia: *Arg.n.*
Depression: *Gels.*, *Ign.*
Emotional: *Ign.*, *Lyc.*
Excitement: (often brings on bilious troubles): *Cham.*
Fear of crowds: *Arg.n.*
    before an event: *Arg.n.*
    of falling: *Gels.*
    of heights: *Arg.n.*
    from shock: *Ign.*
    from strain: *Ign.*
    of water: *Arg.n.*
Impatience: *Acon.*
Intolerance of everything: *Cham.*
    of music: *Acon.*
    of noise: *Acon.*
    of pain: *Acon.*
Irritable: *Ign.*, *Lyc.*
Listless, cannot make an effort: *Gels.*

Moods change rapidly: *Ign*.
Quarrelsome: *Nux.v*.
Restlessness: *Cham*.
Sensitive: *Nux.v*.
Tearful: *Lyc*.
Temper bad: *Cham*.
Tense: *Nux.v*.
Thoughts confused: *Acon*.

Skin Troubles

Boils: *Hep.s., Sil*.
Injury – every little suppurates: *Hep.s., Sil*.
Pain sharp: *Hep.s*.
Sensitive cold sores: *Hep.s*.
Sensitive to touch: *Hep.s*.
Sores which fester: *Hep.s*.
Unhealthy: *Hep.s*.
Worse cold air: *Hep.s*.

Stomach Troubles

Appetite lost when overworked: *Calc.c*.
Assimilation of food poor: *Sil*.
Belching: *Phos*.
      which does not relieve: *Arg.n*.
      frequent, sour: *Calc.c*.
Biliousness: *Bry*.
Bloated feeling: *Puls*.
Colic: *Cham*.
    worse heat: *Bry*.
    worse movement: *Bry*.
    worse pressure: *Bry*.
Craves Cold drinks: *Calc.c., Sil*.
      Cold food: *Sil*.
      Eggs: *Calc.c*.
      Ice-cream: *Sil*.
      Indigestible things: *Calc.c*.
      Salt: *Nat.m*.
      Sweets: *Arg.n., Calc.c., Lyc., Sulph*.

Drinking causes shudders: *Caps.*
Faintness on attempting to sit up: *Bry.*
Food, worse soon after: *Bry.*
Hearburn: *Bry.*
Hunger soon after eating: *Phos.*
Nausea on attempting to sit up: *Bry.*
Pains – burning: *Caps., Puls.*
      burning soon after food: *Ars.alb.*
      Colicky on attempting to eat: *Calc.p.*
      Eating, soon after: *Puls.*
      Worse cold food: *Phos.*
      Worse ice-cream: *Phos.*
Ptomaine poisoning: *Ars.alb.*
Taste sour: *Phos.*
Thirst for cold drinks: *Calc.c.*
      Great, drinks much but small quantities often: *Ars.alb.*
      for large quantities: *Bry.*
      Much: *Caps.*
      None: *Puls.*
      Unquenchable: *Nat.m.*
Vomiting with continuous nausea: *Ant.t.*
      continuous with diarrhoea: *Ant.t.*
      easily: *Calc.p.*
      from fright: *Acon.*
      green, tough, watery: *Ant.t.*
      with violent straining and sweat on forehead: *Ant.t.*
      warm drinks: *Bry.*
      water as soon as warm in stomach: *Phos.*
      with retching: *Ars.alb.*
      with retching and exhaustion and coldness: *Ars.alb.*
Waterbrash: *Bry.*
Wind, better hot applications: *Cham.*
Wind, from bursting feeling: *Arg.n.*

Better after vomiting: *Ars.alb.*
      warm drinks: *Ars.alb.*

Worse food, fat: *Puls.*
      rich: *Puls.*
      sight of: *Ars.alb.*

Worse food, smell of: *Ars.alb.*
Worse Milk: *Sulph.*
Worse Over-eating: *Ant.c., Nux.v.*
Worse Salt, too much: *Phos.*
Worse 11 a.m. wants a snack: *Sulph.*

Sunstroke
Face burning: *Bell.*
  dry: *Bell.*
  hot: *Bell.*
Pulse strong: *Bell.*
Pupils dilated: *Bell.*

Throat Troubles
Adenoids: *Calc.c., Calc.p.*
Colds settle in throat: *Calc.p., Sil.*
Colds bring on tonsillitis: *Calc.p.*
Constricted: *Bell.*
Desires cold water: *Acon.*
Dryness: *Acon., Bell.*
Dryness with thirst: *Lyc.*
Exposure to dry, cold wind: *Acon.*
Glands enlarged: *Calc.c., Calc.p., Sil.*
Hawking of mucus: *Arg.n., Calc.c.*
Hoarseness: *Caust.*
Inflammation: *Lyc.*
   with stitches on swallowing: *Calc.c., Merc., Sil.*
   tonsils: *Bar.c., Bell., Ign.*
   every change of weather: *Merc.*
Mucus: *Caust.*
  Back of throat: *Bar.c.*
  tenacious: *Arg.n.*
  thick: *Arg.n.*
Pain burning: *Acon., Bell., Caust., Merc.*
  pricking, in tonsils: *Sil.*
  raw: *Arg.n., Bell., Caust., Merc.*
  raw in larynx: *Caust.*
  shooting on swallowing: *Caust.*

Pain shooting from throat to ear: *Hep.s.*
  sore: *Arg.n., Bell., Caust., Ign., Merc.*
  sore only when not swallowing: *Caps.*
  sore larynx: *Caust.*
  sore ulcers: *Ign.*
  smarting: *Bar.c., Merc.*
  stitching on swallowing: *Calc.c., Merc., Sil.*
  tingling: *Acon.*
  extending to ears: *Caps.*
  on swallowing: *Acon.*
  in larynx on swallowing: *Hep.s.*
Red: *Bell.*
Red tonsils: *Bell.*
Sensation of crumb in: *Hep.s.*
   of splinter on swallowing: *Arg.n.*
   of plug in throat: *Bar.c.*
Sensitive to draughts: *Hep.s.*
  externally: *Hep.s.*
  internally: *Hep.s.*
Suppuration of tonsils: *Bar.c., Lyc.*
Swallow, constant urging: *Bell.*
Swallowing difficult: *Calc.c.*
    worse liquids: *Bar.c.*
Swelling of tonsils: *Bar.c., Calc.c., Calc.p.*
Symptoms from right to left: *Lyc.*
Ulcers: *Merc.*
Ulceration of tonsils: *Lyc.*
Uvula dark red: *Arg.n.*
Voice lost: *Caust., Merc.*
  rough: *Arg.n., Caust.*

Better warm drinks: *Lyc.*

Worse evening: *Acon.*
  night: *Bell.*
Worse around midnight: *Acon.*
  cold drinks: *Lyc.*

Toothache
Gumboil: *Bell.*

Gums bleed easily: *Hep.s.*
Mouth dry: *Puls.*
Pain after fillings: *Acon.*
Pain great: *Puls.*
Sensitive, very: *Hep.s.*
Throbbing with dry mouth: *Bell.*
Worse cold water: *Puls.*
      heat: *Puls.*
      hot fluids: *Puls.*

Urination
Urinating, child may cry before: *Lyc.*
      delay in starting: *Lyc.*
Urine increase at night: *Lyc.*
      red sediment in: *Lyc.*

Whooping Cough
After drinking: *Ant.t., Bry.*
After eating: *Ant.t., Bry.*
Cries before cough starts: *Ant.t., Bell.*
Dry: *Bry.*
Dry throat: *Bell.*
Mucus, large amounts vomited: *Ant.t.*
      cannot be raised: *Ant.t.*
      Rattling: *Ant.t.*
Spasms until mucus is raised: *Bell.*
Vomits then returns to finish meal: *Bry.*
With nausea: *Ant.t.*
With nose-bleeds: *Merc.*
With stomach pains: *Bell.*
With Cold sweat on forehead: *Ant.t.*
When a flow of tears with cough: *Nat.m.*
When getting warm in bed: *Ant.t.*

Wounds
Bleed easily even if small: *Phos.*

THE 25 REMEDIES AND ABBREVIATIONS

Aconitum Napellus	Acon.
Antimonium Crudum	Ant. c.
Antimonium Tartaricum	Ant. t.
Argentum Nitricum	Arg. n.
Arsenicum Album	Ars. alb.
Baryta Carb	Bar. c.
Belladonna	Bell.
Bryonia	Bry.
Calcarea Carbonica	Calc. c.
Calcarea Phosphorica	Calc. p.
Capsicum	Caps.
Causticum	Caust.
Chamomilla	Cham.
Cinchona Officinalis	China.
Gelsemium	Gels.
Hepar Sulphuris	Hep. s.
Ignatia	Ign.
Lycopodium	Lyc.
Mercurius	Merc.
Natrum Muriaticum	Nat.m.
Nux Vomica	Nux. v.
Phosphorus	Phos.
Pulsatilla	Puls.
Silicea	Sil.
Sulphur	Sulph.

BOOKS FOR FURTHER READING AND STUDY

Arnica by Phyllis Speight, pub. by Health Science Press.
Homoeopathy in Epidemic Diseases by Dr. Dorothy Shepherd, pub. by Health Science Press.
Homoeopathy, First Aid (in accidents and ailments) by Dr. D. M. Gibson, pub. by The British Homoeopathic Association.
Homoeopathy and Immunization by Leslie J. Speight, pub. by Health Science Press.
Homoeopathy – A Practical Guide to Natural Medicine by Phyllis Speight, pub. by Granada Publishing Company.
Pointers to the Common Remedies by Tyler and Borland Nos. 1, 2 and 5, pub. by The British Homoeopathic Association.

HOMOEOPATHIC CHEMISTS

Ainsworth's Homoeopathic Pharmacy, 38 New Cavendish Street, London, W1M 7LH.
Galen Homoeopathics, Lewell Mill, Dorchester, Dorset DT2 8AN.
A. Nelson & Co. Ltd, 5 Endeavour Way, Wimbledon, London, SW19 9UH.
E. Gould & Son Ltd, 14 Crowndale Road, London NW1 1TT.
The above all have a good postal service.

HOMOEOPATHIC HOSPITALS

The Royal London Homoeopathic Hospital, Great Ormond Street, London, WC1N 3HR.
Glasgow Homoeopathic Hospital, 1000 Great Western Road, Glasgow, C12.
Bristol Homoeopathic Hospital, Cotham, Bristol 6.
Tunbridge Wells Homoeopathic Hospital, Church Road, Tunbridge Wells, Kent.
All in the National Health Service.

The British Homoeopathic Association, 27a Devonshire Street, London, W1N 1RJ.